Hoof Care for Horses

Henry Heymering, C.J.F., R.M.F.

CONTENTS

Introduction

When it comes to caring for your horse, good advice never goes out-of-date. In 380 B.C., Xenophon, the Greek general and author of *On Horsemanship,* wrote of the importance of making sure a horse's feet are dry: "Washing down of the legs is a thing I absolutely forbid; it does no good — on the contrary, daily washing is bad for the hooves." He also noted, "Even naturally sound hooves get spoiled in stalls with moist, smooth [flat] floors. The floors should be sloping to avoid moisture. . . . The mere standing on such [completely dry] floors strengthens the feet." As Xenophon was responsible for at least one 3,000-mile military excursion on horseback, his recommendations can be trusted, and they still ring true today.

The requirements for maintaining healthy hooves are the same as for maintaining a horse in overall good health: a clean and dry environment with good diet and sufficient exercise, and regular care from a qualified professional. Any problems with a horse's hooves will have an immediate and serious impact on his health and usefulness. There is an old saying that is as true today as it ever was: "No foot, no horse."

Prevention Comes First

Preventive maintenance will do more to improve hoof health than any and all corrective treatments, and it will prove to be less expensive. The most important requirements are dry footing, good ventilation, proper diet, and exercise.

Dry Footing

A common misconception in hoof care is the idea that hooves regularly require external moisture — moisturizing dressings or mud or water to stand in. On the contrary, knowledgeable horsemen have long stressed the importance of keeping the hooves dry. Even a small amount of outside moisture may prove to be excessive; horses with dry feet will be much easier to keep healthy. To ensure that your horse's feet are clean and dry, you must properly maintain all of the locations where you keep him.

To Shoe or Not to Shoe?

Free-roaming "wild" horses do fine without shoes, as do brood mares, so why should horses be shod? There are three reasons to shoe horses: protection, traction, and support for the leg. If none of these reasons apply, then your horse does not need shoes.

- **Protection.** Shoes lessen hoof wear and help prevent cracking and chipping. Excessive wear usually comes from improper management — hooves that are too soft and weak from moisture and urine cannot stand much use.
- **Traction.** With shoes, traction can be modified according to riding discipline or use. Horses that pull wagons or logs want more traction — as much as possible. Reining horses to do a sliding stop requires less than normal traction.
- **Support.** With shoes (or, for foals, sometimes with artificial hoof material such as Equilox, Grand Circuit, or Equithane), the area the horse stands on can be extended to provide more support. A foal that stands base-wide, for example, can be fitted with shoes that put the area contacting the ground more directly under the leg. A horse with a bowed tendon, a strained suspensory ligament, or with navicular disease may be shod with a shoe that extends behind the heels of the hoof to provide more support to the leg and decrease tendon and ligament strain.

Stalls. The stall floor should be higher than the surrounding ground, slightly inclined, and impermeable so that the flooring doesn't collect or retain moisture, especially urine. Clay is an excellent material for flooring; once it is packed down, it stays separate from the bedding, prevents urine from soaking in, and provides some cushioning. Solid rubber mats, which are available commercially for stall flooring, work even better and can be installed over any fairly smooth surface. Any dry bedding is adequate if the dampened and soiled bedding is removed at least once a day and the floor allowed to completely air-dry. If any urine is left to soak into the flooring, the stall eventually becomes an open latrine. Sprinkling lime (the slaked or hydrated type) or a commercial product like Sweet PDZ over the bare floor at least once a week before bedding down will reduce odors and eliminate many disease-causing organisms.

Paddocks and loafing sheds. Small areas such as these encourage horses to stand in their own urine and manure, and the ammonia from these is even more destructive to hooves than is the moisture. Manure in paddocks and loafing sheds should be picked up every day. Horses tend to avoid urinating on hard surfaces that would cause the urine to splash on their own legs; this means that if hay is fed on the ground, the horses will trample some hay underfoot and urinate on it, then stand in that area. You can prevent this by keeping the hay off the ground or by feeding it from hayracks with mats underneath. To further discourage horses from urinating where they loaf, lay down smooth rubber mats without bedding or hay in the areas they most often stand, and put down a little old bedding or hay in a different area for urination.

Pastures. As with paddocks, ensure that horses do not loaf in their pasture bathroom areas. Filling potholes and draining swampy areas of the pasture — and fencing off those areas until repairs are completed — will keep your horse's hooves drier; it will also help to control mosquitoes and horseflies.

Ventilation

Without adequate ventilation, floors will not air-dry, and ammonia from urine left on floors will collect. Ammonia on the floor dissolves hooves, and the presence of ammonia in the stall air has been linked to pneumonia in foals. A horse may generate 10 gallons of moisture — through its urine and exhaled moisture — each day. Outlet vents must be installed to remove the old moist air, and inlet vents must be installed to supply fresh clean air.

As the air in the stall warms, it holds more moisture and naturally rises, so roof outlet vents such as turbines, cupolas, or ridge vents will provide escape for the foul air. The total size of these outlets needs to equal about 1 to 1½ percent of the area of the floor. For example, a 20-foot-by-20-foot building has a floor area of 400 square feet and would need 4 to 6 square feet of outlet vent, such as a ridge vent 10 feet long with a 6-inch throat.

Inlet air vents must cover two to three times as much area as the outlets. They should be larger, more widely spaced, and located above horses to reduce drafts.

Proper Diet

Environmental factors such as dry footing and adequate ventilation have by far the most influence on the health and integrity of the hoof, but good nutrition also plays a role. A horse's diet should be mostly grass or grass hay, supplemented with a loose salt-mineral mix, with plenty of fresh water. The healthiest working ranch horses I've seen ate nothing more than grass and loose salt-mineral.

A salt-mineral supplement is necessary because of the declining mineral content of our soils; grass and hays alone no longer provide sufficient minerals for horses. A loose salt-mineral mix (such as MoorMan's GroStrong or similar products by Carnation or Purina) can be fed free-choice and is generally palatable, inexpensive, and effective. A loose salt-mineral is superior to trace-mineral salt blocks because it contains not only salt and trace minerals but also major minerals (such as calcium and phosphorus) and vitamins.

Exercise

Daily exercise is important to maintain blood circulation and the health of the hooves. Free-roaming horses will travel 20 to 30 miles per day, so for domestic horses it is impossible to overdo walking or mild exercise — the more, the better.

Traveling on Shoes of Iron

The first record of iron horseshoes can be found in a 910 A.D. account by Emperor Leo VI. By the time of the Crusades (1096–1270), horse shoeing was popular all across Europe. Shoes not only protected the horses' feet but also gave the knights a psychological advantage. What a fearsome sight it must have been to see an armored rider charging with sparks flying from his horse's feet!

In the centuries since, armies on horseback have always relied on horseshoes. The Spanish explorer Juan de Onante's 1598 expedition to America carried 5,256 spare horseshoes! And during the Civil War, one key to the Union's success was that only the northern states had any horseshoe-making machines.

Dietary Supplements for Good Hoof Health

In addition to a loose salt-mineral, other supplements to your horse's diet can help prevent hoof problems and promote good overall health.

Supplement	Benefits
Vitamin A	The vitamin most commonly found to be deficient in horses. A deficiency of vitamin A may cause the hoof horn to be brittle and unevenly laid down. A supplement of about 100,000 IU of vitamin A per day should correct any deficiency and is also safe for horses that are not deficient. Signs that indicate a vitamin A deficiency include perioples that look like fish scales, a slowness to completely shed out in spring, shivering in cold weather, white line disease, scratches, rain rot, a rough coat, or an inability to sweat.
Biotin	Ordinarily produced in sufficient quantity in the horse's gut. However, some horses under stress may have a deficiency, which can result in weak hooves or a poor coat. Biotin is not toxic, so you can safely try 30 mg per day for a few months. In my experience, however, biotin makes a noticeable improvement in hooves for only about one horse in every twenty. If you don't see an improvement in 4 to 5 months, discontinue the biotin.
Flaxseed meal	A good source of omega-3 fatty acids, which are very beneficial anti-inflammatory substances. Adding half a cup of flaxseed meal a day to feed can help put a healthy shine on coats and hooves. This is a good supplement for all horses, but especially those with dull coats, allergies, or arthritis.
Grains (concentrates)	Necessary only when a horse uses more energy than he can get from the amount of grass or hay he can eat. A common misconception is that concentrated feeds are "complete" and will meet all of a horse's nutritional requirements. Concentrated feeds are complete in terms of offering the right percentages of necessary nutrients, but not in terms of amounts. In other words, if your horse normally eats

Supplement	Benefits
Grains *(cont'd.)* (concentrates)	15 pounds of grass and hay a day, he would have to eat a full 15 pounds of commercial grain mix in a day to receive the recommended minimums for all minerals and vitamins. However, he would then have a great excess of digestible energy, and his feet would probably develop founder. Commercial grain mixes are intended to be used as an energy supplement, not a total diet.
Iodine	Deficient in grass and hay, though it is sufficiently present in salt and other supplements that a horse is unlikely to develop an iodine deficiency. Iodine is antifungal and may help horses with white line disease.
Protein	Needs to make up only about 10 percent of the diet for most adult horses not in heavy work. Excess nitrogen from too much protein and/or alfalfa hay causes an increase in ammonia in the urine. Horses with slow hoof growth may benefit from increasing protein up to 14 percent.
Selenium	Similar to iodine in the amount that is needed and the amount that is toxic, and also like iodine, it is antifungal and is typically deficient in the ration. However, unlike iodine, selenium is not present in sufficient quantities in most supplements. Most horses benefit from an additional 1 to 2 mg per day of selenium. You should certainly supplement selenium if your horse shows any signs of deficiency — yellow frogs, allergies, dull coat, and sore suspensory ligaments — or if he is used in any work or athletic sport. Early reversible signs of selenium toxicity are mane and tail hairs falling out. If you live west of the Mississippi River or you have concerns about toxicity, have your vet perform a blood test before providing additional selenium.
Zinc	Has been shown to improve hoof quality in cattle and is likely to help horses as well. Toxicity is rare.

A Hoof Care Glossary

In order to understand what hoof care your horse may need and what problems can arise, it helps to know the proper terms for the various parts and landmarks of the hoof.

Buttresses or bars. Buttresses, also called bars, are the continuations of the wall, visible from the bottom of the hoof, that run forward from the heels towards the point of the frog. The buttresses help strengthen and stabilize the hoof wall at the heels and provide the outer boundary for the collateral sulci.

Center of rotation. The center of rotation is the center of hoof balance in a standing horse. It is located near the lower end of the short pastern bone. As the horse is standing, a line directly below that center of rotation would fall to a point about one-third the length of the frog back from the point of the frog.

Coffin bone. The coffin bone is so named because it rests in a hard box (the hoof wall) that is lined with softer cushioning material (the laminae), much like a body in a coffin or a violin in its case. The coffin bone is also called the P3 or third phalanx. It is the main bone inside the hoof, and the wall is attached to it.

Coffin joint. The coffin joint is the joint between the coffin bone, the short pastern bone, and the navicular bone.

Collateral sulci. On either side of the frog are grooves called the collateral sulci. These allow the frog to expand in response to pressure, thereby dissipating rather than transmitting the pressure from the ground and protecting the deep digital flexor tendon, which is above the frog.

Coronary band. The coronary band is the soft tissue at the top of the hoof wall, underneath the periople, from which the hoof wall is produced.

Coronet. The upper exterior border of the hoof wall is called the coronet.

Duckett's dot. This is a point about 3/8 inch behind the tip of the frog. It is directly below the spot where the deep digital flexor tendon and the extensor tendon attach to the coffin bone. Duckett's dot is the center of the radius of the tip of the coffin bone.

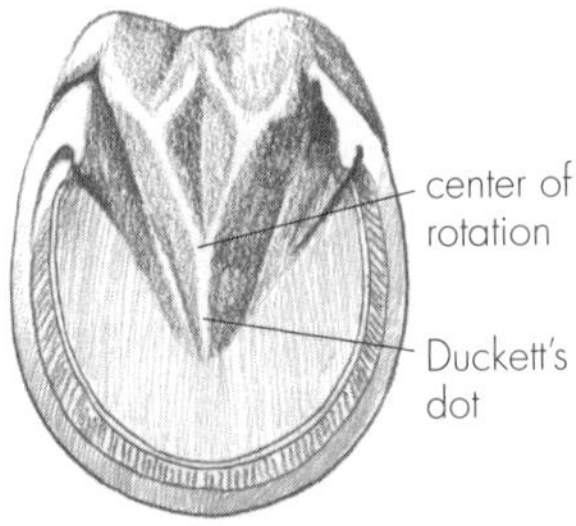

Knowing where Duckett's dot and the center of rotation are helps you find the point of breakover on a horse's toe.

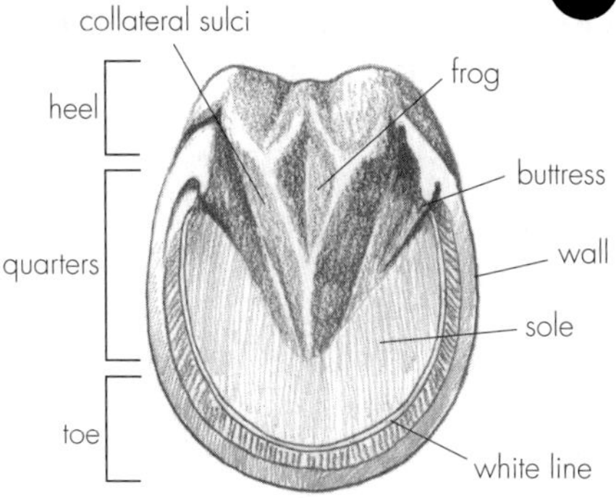

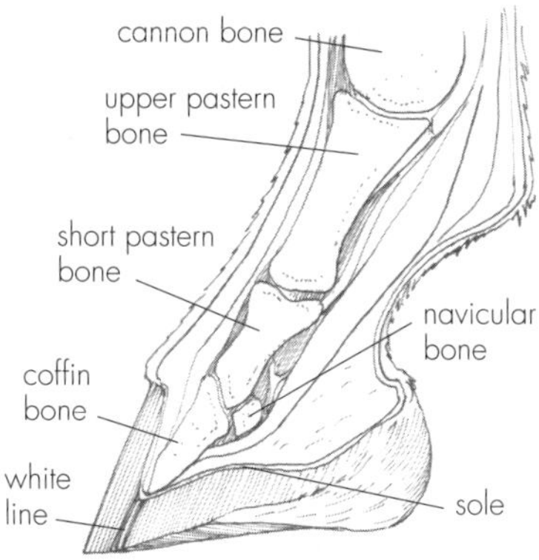

Fetlock hairs. Far from being an unnecessary decoration, fetlock hairs or "feathers" serve the very useful function of keeping excess water away from the hoof. Watch a horse with fetlock hairs being bathed and you will see the water run down its legs and then straight down the fetlock hairs and away from the hoof, just like a drain pipe.

Frog. The rubbery, triangular-shaped part on the bottom of the hoof is the frog. Like the wall and the sole, the frog is composed of both tubules and intertubular horn. However, the frog has a moisture content of about 50 percent, which is higher than that of the wall or sole, and it contains a large amount of fat. The frog is perfectly designed and situated to prevent pressure from the ground from affecting the deep digital flexor tendon, which runs directly above the frog.

Laminae. The laminae (also called lamellum) are complex vertical corrugations or leaves in the hoof. The sensitive (or dermal) laminae that attach to the coffin bone interleave with the horny (or epidermal) laminae that form the inner part of the hoof wall. This intricate dovetailing allows the body weight to be transferred from the bony column to the hoof wall, and it also allows the hoof wall to slide down past the coffin bone as the hoof wall grows out. Each hoof contains approximately 650 laminae, and taken all together, they provide about 8 square feet of attachment per hoof.

Navicular bone. The navicular bone is a small canoe-shaped bone that forms the lower rear half of the coffin joint. The navicular bone acts like a pulley to keep the deep digital flexor tendon stable in its attachment to the coffin bone. It also provides some cushioning to the coffin joint.

Periople. The periople is the raised soft tissue at the top of the hoof wall that helps protect the coronary band. It usually is about ¾-inch wide. When soaked in water, the periople becomes puffy and milky-colored; after it dries out, it will look pockmarked.

Quarters. The quarters of the wall are the portions of the hoof wall between the toe and the heels. The sharper radius at the transition from the toe area to the quarters is called the "toe quarter," and the transition from the quarters to the heel is called the "heel quarter."

Sole. The sole covers the majority of the bottom of the hoof. With 30 percent moisture, the sole is slightly moister than the hoof wall and slightly less moist than the frog. The sole covers and protects the bottom of the coffin bone.

Stratum tectorium. Also called the "hoof varnish," this is a very thin, clear layer of tubular horn on the outside of the hoof wall that helps shed water and keep the hoof dry.

Wall. The hoof wall is the external hard encasement for the hoof. It is composed of parallel vertical hairlike tubules bound together with intertubular horn. The moisture content of the wall averages about 25 percent but has a natural gradient from the outside (15 percent) to the inside (40 percent). This serves to make the hoof harder and tougher on the outside and softer and more cushioning on the inside. All necessary moisture is supplied by the interior of the hoof, and any external moisture will imbalance this gradient.

White line. The white line is the continuation of the horny laminae that joins the sole to the wall; it is visible on the bottom of the hoof. It is the most porous part of the hoof wall, making it more susceptible to infection and the most likely location for an abscess. The white line is used by farriers as a guide to proper placement of the horseshoe nails. Though called "white," this line is actually typically yellowish and should not be confused with the white, unpigmented inner third of the hoof wall.

Home Hoof Care: Cleaning Hooves

Most hoof care, such as trimming and shoeing, should be done by a professional, but one task that every horse owner must do regularly is cleaning hooves. Cleaning the hooves should be part of your routine whenever you groom your horse. Hooves should also be picked out both before and immediately after riding to prevent you from riding or putting away a horse whose hoof has a stone or other hard object wedged in it.

While you're cleaning hooves, check for bent or loose shoes and popped clinches (clinches that stick up from the hoof wall), and look for signs of any of the common hoof problems listed on pages 20 to 31.

The Right Way to Pick Up a Hoof

The first part of this job is learning how to pick up the foot correctly. A common mistake when picking up a horse's foot is pushing against the horse to unweight his leg and then pulling the foot up — this teaches the horse to lean on you. To teach the horse to pick up his foot on his own, without leaning on you, simply use your fingernail to pinch the skin against the cannon bone. Reflexively, as if a fly had landed on his leg, the horse will pick up his foot. Start with very light pressure and wait a few seconds for this response; if there is none, increase the pressure and wait again. The instant the horse starts to pick up his foot, release the pressure immediately, and hold the foot by the tip of the toe. Allow the horse to move his leg wherever he wants — if you wrestle with him, you will only be teaching him that wrestling is acceptable. However, if you keep the toe up, he will not put his foot down.

How to Clean the Hoof

To clean the hoof, gently insert the tip of a hoof pick on either side of the back of the frog under the dirt. The majority of packed-in dirt should easily pop out with a flick of your wrist. The remainder of the dirt can then be scraped out with the pick and/or a hoof brush. When you have cleaned out the hoof, put your horse's foot down gently on the ground and pet him.

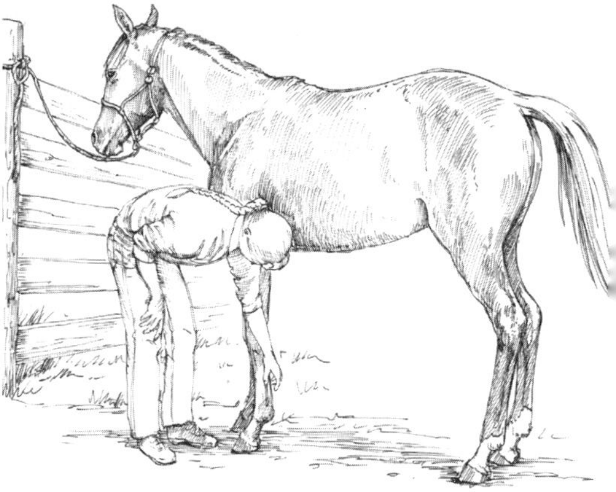

To get a horse to pick up his foot, run your hand down his leg and pinch the skin against the cannon bone.

Finding a Good Hoof Care Professional

A hoof care professional can help you get maximum performance and longevity from your horse. To get quality horseshoeing, trimming, and other hoof care work, however, you need to know what qualifications your hoof care professional should have and how to recognize proper hoof care work.

I use the term "hoof care professional" to include all those who work on horses' feet. Whether you call them shoers, farriers, blacksmiths, trimmers, or hoof care specialists (a term that usually refers to anti-shoeing trimmers), the same basic requirements apply — knowledge, skill, and years of experience.

(Note: I use the masculine pronoun in reference to hoof care professionals simply because the majority of them are men. This is in no way meant to overlook the many women who are excellent hoof care professionals.)

Five Essential Qualities in a Hoof Care Professional

1. The horses he has been trimming or shoeing like him.

Watch a hoof care professional trim or shoe several horses that he has been attending regularly. Horses know when they are being helped or hindered. The horses' attitude toward the hoof care professional will tell you a great deal.

2. He has at least four years of experience.

Consider four years of full-time professional hoof care experience a minimum before you let someone work on your horse, unless he is an apprentice under the supervision of a master. Shoeing and trimming cannot be learned from a book. It takes years for a hoof care professional to begin to truly see the effects of what he is doing. If a hoof care professional has less than four years of experience, let him learn on someone else's horses.

3. He expresses a real concern and interest in your horse, how he moves, and whether he has any problems.

A good hoof care professional cares about how the horse functions. He'll want to see your horses move and ask for your concerns.

4. He has an ability to handle horses well and an obvious delight in his work and in horses.

To be a good hoof care professional, one must know horses very well and be able to tell the difference between a horse that is misbehaving because of pain or fear and one that is acting out because of lack of discipline. (Most often, misbehavior is caused by pain or fear.) Discipline may need to be administered, but never in a way that hurts the horse.

5. He is honest and forthright.

Driving a nail into the quick happens rarely, but it does happen — because of faulty nails, inconsistent hoof walls, the horse suddenly moving, or a mistake. If your hoof care professional tells you about it, you can treat the puncture wound, get a tetanus booster for the horse, and keep the hoof clean and dry for a few days. If he doesn't tell you, it could turn into a big problem. Your hoof care professional should also be willing to say "I don't know" and to seek help or refer you to another specialist if necessary.

Special Qualifications for Hoof Care Professionals

The qualifications above are the basic requirements for any hoof care professional. However, if you have a foal, a performance horse, or a horse with any lameness problems, you will need a hoof care professional with greater expertise.

- **More experience.** For the above situations, a hoof care professional should have 10 years or more experience — the more the better. A professional with 10 years experience has had the opportunity to see the effects of trimming and shoeing on the athletic career of some horses and has been able to watch the longer progression of chronic diseases like founder and navicular disease.

- **Continuing education.** A performance and/or therapeutic hoof care professional should read the professional journals and attend clinics and seminars. He should be a member of state and national farrier associations. One can never know it all.

How to Keep a Good Hoof Care Professional

Hanging on to a good hoof care professional is every bit as important as finding one. A professional can do a better job for you and your horses if he is familiar with them and their history. Once you've found a good professional, work to keep him by doing the following:

- **Respect the professional's time.** Have your horses caught and ready, with clean dry legs and picked-out hooves.
- **Respect the professional's expertise.** If you've done your homework and found an experienced, knowledgeable hoof care professional, you should follow his advice. Do not tell him how to do his job. You are paying for his expertise, and if you can't trust him, then stop wasting your money and his time — get a better hoof care professional, one you respect.
- **Stick around.** Be there to ask and answer questions, walk or jog the horse for him, and discuss any problems. Pay him immediately when he's done, and make arrangements for the next appointment. Let him know whenever there is a problem that might be related to hoof care.
- **Provide a good place to work.** The shoeing area should be clean, accessible, level, protected from the weather, well lit (preferably lit from the sides to eliminate shadows), uncramped, safe, and free from traffic, obstructions, and distractions. Dogs and children should not be playing underfoot.
- **Make sure your horses are cooperative.** Your hoof care professional may not be able to do quality work on an uncooperative horse. If he recommends that you have your horse trained professionally or that your vet tranquilize the horse, then have that done.
- **Keep a regular schedule.** Have your horses' hooves attended to on a four- to eight- week schedule, as your hoof care professional recommends. Make appointments well in advance, and keep them.

- **Certification by the American Farriers Association (AFA) and/or the Guild of Professional Farriers (GPF).** This certification should be at least the Basic AFA Certification (CF) and preferably AFA Journeyman Certification (CJF) — the AFA's current top level — or GPF Registered Journeyman Farrier (RJF). These journeyman tests require extensive knowledge of anatomy and shoeing as well as forge work. These associations list certified members on their Web sites: www.amfarriers.com and www.horseshoes.com/theguild.
- **Teaching and/or researching.** A still higher level of qualification would include those who write, research, lecture, or teach shoeing. A Registered Master Farrier (RMF) of the Guild of Professional Farriers meets these additional criteria.

Holding a Horse During Shoeing or Trimming

For shoeing or trimming to be a pleasant experience for all involved, a horse needs to be held in a way that makes him comfortable and cooperative. He should not be expecting to eat (if it is his normal meal time, feed him first). If the horse is emotionally attached to another horse, that horse should be kept in sight. If you are bringing the horse in directly from the pasture, you should put him in a stall for a few minutes or give him some other opportunity to urinate before having to stand for a long time.

Check with your hoof care professional first if you intend to cover your horse with fly repellent before a shoeing or trimming; some hoof care professionals and veterinarians are allergic to fly repellents. Shade, fans, and fly whisks can be used instead of sprays to keep flies away. Don't apply hoof dressings before shoeing, as they gum up rasps and make the hooves slippery. The horse's legs should be clean and dry.

The following directions are fairly universal; however, if your hoof care professional prefers something different, follow his requests — he is the one under the horse holding sharp tools in his hands.

Rope or Chain?

Hold the horse's lead rope at least 2 feet from the snap with slack in the rope. Horses are more quiet and comfortable when they are less restricted. However, the horse should not be allowed to move from the spot where he's standing. Any attempt by the horse to move from the spot should be blocked. If the horse manages to move he should be immediately put back in the original spot by the most direct route.

If the horse has a tendency to move, or especially to walk over you, then a chain over the nose is helpful. I prefer an 8-foot length of 1-inch cotton rope attached to a 30-inch chain. The chain should go through the ring on the left side of the horse's halter from outside to inside; go up; then down across the nose on top of the nose band; then through the ring on the right side of the halter from inside to outside; and then attach to the ring on the right side of the halter just below the ear. In this way the chain rests on the halter's nose piece and not directly on the horse. The chain need only be shaken or rattled to be effective. You should never yank on the chain, and you should never tie a horse with a chain over his nose.

Horses that can be tied for shoeing or trimming should be tied with a rope that ties to a loop of baling twine at the wall (or walls), so that if the horse panics he will not injure himself fighting the ties, and when the baling twine breaks there will still be a rope attached to his halter. Elastic ties can snap and seriously injure an eye.

Reprimanding a Horse

In general, never hit a horse while the hoof care professional is underneath the horse. Typically, when you hit or startle a horse or shank him with the nose chain he will slam his foot to the ground. This is not a good thing when the hoof care professional is holding that foot. The one exception to this rule seems to be when a "dogging bat" (two wide strips of leather about 18-inch-long sewn together, available at Western tack stores) is used. For me, it is the only thing a holder can safely use to reprimand a horse while I'm underneath it.

Where Is the Best Place to Stand?

When the hoof care professional is working on a front foot, you should stand at the horse's opposite shoulder. You will be safely out of the way should the horse pull his foot away and paw. Should the horse rear or panic in any way, your natural reaction is to back up — when you do that you will be pulling the horse away from (rather than on top of) the professional.

When the professional is working on a hind foot, you should stand at the horse's shoulder on the same side. If the horse panics your natural reaction will be to back up, which will swing the horse's hind end away from you and the professional.

Are Tranquilizers Necessary?

Tranquilizers are a poor substitute for proper handling and training of the horse, but occasionally they may be necessary. They should only be administered by a veterinarian. In my experience, acepromazine and Rompun do not discourage horses from kicking but may actually make it more likely that they will kick because they remove the horse's inhibitions. Additionally, tranquilizers seem to take away the horse's awareness and ability to learn from the experience. The only tranquilizer that I've found safe for trimming or shoeing is Dormosedan (detomidine hydrochloride).

Evaluating a Trimming or Shoeing Job

The easiest and most common way for an owner to judge a trimming or shoeing job is by whether it looks neat and pretty and whether the shoes stay on. Veterinarians are typically more concerned with hoof balance, and they may measure for equal heel lengths. Trainers often look for performance results, even at the expense of long-term soundness.

Unfortunately, each one of those criteria may be misleading, and even all of them put together may not guarantee that your horse will be properly trimmed or shoed. A quality job is one that allows the horse to function well and maintain soundness. Keep in mind also that the only fair time to judge a trimming or shoeing job is right after it is done, not weeks or months later. In addition, remember that:

- The most functional job is not necessarily the most attractive.
- When a shoe is lost, it is usually because of factors other than the quality of the shoeing job.
- A horse's balance is not determined by whether the heels have equal height.
- Future soundness does not have to be — and should not be! — sacrificed for temporary performance.

While no rule of thumb can be followed without exception, the following criteria will give you a good indication of the quality of a trimming or shoeing job.

Breakover

The *point of breakover* is the most forward part of the hoof or shoe that the foot pivots over as the heels leave the ground during locomotion. The position of the point of breakover affects the strain on the leg during movement. Duckett's dot is a spot on the frog about ⅜ inch farther back from the toe of the horse's hoof than the point of the frog (see page 8). The distance from Duckett's dot to the outside edge of the wall should be very nearly the same to the right and to the left. Moving that same distance from Duckett's dot to the toe gives you an excellent rule of thumb for the proper position of the breakover at the toe. However, there are exceptions, such as gaited horses and others that can be conditioned to accept the extra strain of a longer breakover point. A faster breakover than normal may be necessary to treat a variety of leg problems such as founder, navicular disease, and bowed tendons. Rockering the toe is one method to bring the point of breakover back. Another method is to simply set the shoe back from the front edge of the toe.

Support

The heels of the shoe should extend back at least ⅛ to ½ inch or more past the ends of the heels of the hoof. The further back the shoe comes, the more support it gives to the flexor tendons and suspensory ligament. To shoe a horse without extending the heels of the shoes behind the heels of the hoof increases the strain compared to an unshod hoof because of increased lever arm — the angle and distance from the fetlock to the point where the heel meets the ground. Contrary to popular belief, most hunter/jumpers, barrel horses, racehorses, and so on will keep shoes like this on without problem. In fact, many horses lose shoes less frequently when they have the heels slightly extended than they do when the shoe heels are flush with the heel of the hoof.

A good rule of thumb for the minimum amount of support needed is that the heels of the hoof or the heels of the shoe should extend as far behind Duckett's dot as the breakover point is in front of it. It is better if the heels are as far behind the center of rotation of the foot as the breakover point extends in front of the center of rotation.

Hoof Shape and Shoe Fit

Providing the hoof is free of damage or defects in the wall, the bottom of the hoof wall should rest flush against the ground or shoe with no gaps visible from the outside. The shoe and bottom edge of the hoof should follow the shape of the coronary band, and ideally the wall should be straight, without flares, from the coronary band to the ground. Existing flares may need to be removed by rasping. The shoe should be slightly wider than the hoof at the heels of the foot; the toe of the shoe may be backed up behind the toe of the hoof in order to facilitate breakover; and the shoe may be placed for support where the wall should be but isn't.

Toe Length

Toe length should be as short as possible while still adequately protecting the sole from bruising on rocks and other hard objects. The sole should not yield to strong thumb pressure, and the hoof wall should be slightly longer than the sole, allowing for some cup to the foot. A typical 1,000-pound horse has about a 3¼-inch toe length for the front foot and a slightly longer one for the hind feet.

Hoof Angle

As a rule of thumb, the hoof angle should match the pastern angle. However, hoof angles lower than 53 degrees put increased strain on the heel of the hoof, cause run-under heels (see page 25) and navicular disease (see page 31), and increase the strain on the flexor tendons — leading to bowed tendons. Hoof angles higher than 60 degrees may be indicative of club foot (see page 29), or they may cause the pastern to drop too far and put excessive strain on the suspensory ligament.

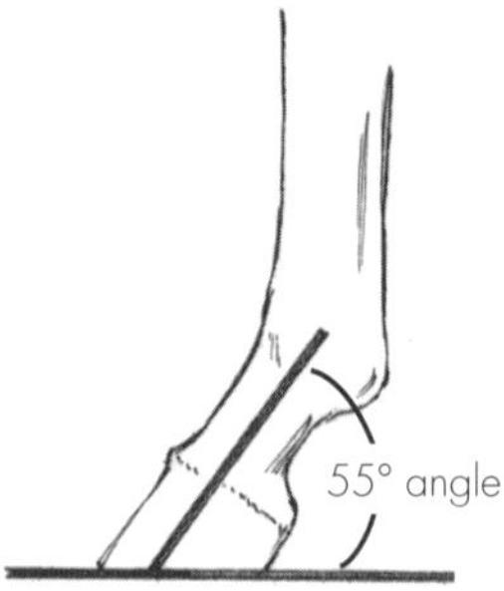

The hoof angles should match the pastern angle.

Hoof Balance

Growth rings on the hoof should be parallel to each other and to the coronet, and both sides of the shoe should wear equally. (Some lame horses will be an exception to this, as will some toed-out horses.) When viewed from the front of the hoof, the grain of the horse's hoof should be straight and perpendicular to the ground. If the grain is at an angle, it indicates that the hoof is out of balance. If the grain is curved, it indicates longstanding balance problems.

Attitude, Posture, Gaits, and Movement

Your horse should move as well or better after being shod than he did just before being shod. He should also stand as well, or even more comfortably and squarely with improved posture. The horse's overall attitude, and especially his attitude as he works, should also be as good or better than before he was trimmed or shod.

Common Shoe Problems

Your hoof care professional is the person who is best qualified to observe your horse, note any hoof problems, and determine the proper remedy. However, these brief suggestions may help you notice and understand the most common problems.

Thrown Shoes

Why do horses throw shoes? A better question might be, How do they keep them on? All it takes to throw a shoe is for the horse to step on the shoe with another of its feet; for the shoe to catch on something (a rock, the edge of a concrete pad, and so on) as the horse is moving; or for the horse to paw and catch the heels of the shoe on something.

Weak or styrofoam-type hooves (see page 25) may not be strong enough to hold shoes. But even assuming the hooves are strong enough, it is not possible to totally prevent shoe loss, and you would not want to if you could. If a shoe is trapped by another hoof or by an object, it is better for the shoe to come off than for the trapped leg to be strained. Methods used to prevent thrown shoes should therefore focus on keeping the shoes from being stepped on or caught rather than on making the shoes more firmly attached. Thick bell boots will deflect other hooves and reduce the chance that a horse will throw a shoe. Clips at the ends of the heels (sometimes called spooned heels) can reduce the chance that the exposed edge will catch on anything. Shortening the length of shoe heel is counterproductive — it reduces the shoe's support and often makes it more likely that the horse will step on a shoe.

Won't Boots Do Instead?

Boots can be used in place of shoes for some horses, especially if protection is just needed for occasional rough terrain. Boots provide protection and traction but not support. They should not be used for more than a few hours at a time, because, much like rubber gloves, boots tend to trap moisture.

Bent or Twisted Shoes

You should have some basic tools on hand (rasp, crease nail pullers, pull-offs) in case you need to remove a bent, twisted, or loose shoe (for example, when duct tape won't keep the shoe on until your farrier can come to remove it, or when the shoe is sufficiently mangled that it is unsafe to keep on). First use the smooth side of an old farrier's rasp to carefully file off the clinches (the folded-over shank of the horseshoe nails where they exit the wall), then use a nail to clean dirt away from the heads of the nails. Next, use a crease nail puller to pull one nail at a time (especially if the foot is sore or weak) and finally shoe pullers to gently pry off the shoe if there are any nails remaining that could not be removed.

Have your farrier show you how to remove a shoe when he's working on your horse for a regular appointment — before you have an emergency.

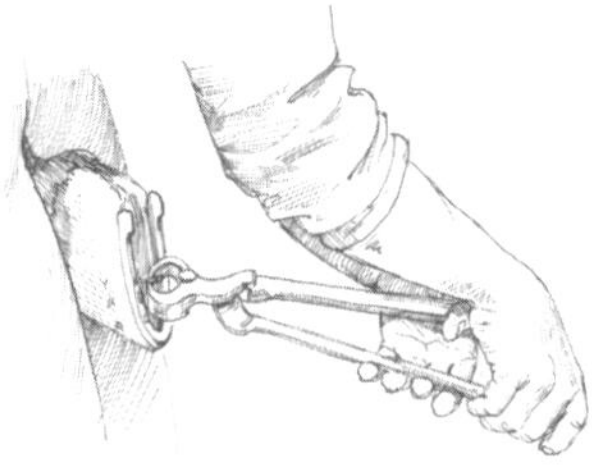

Step 1

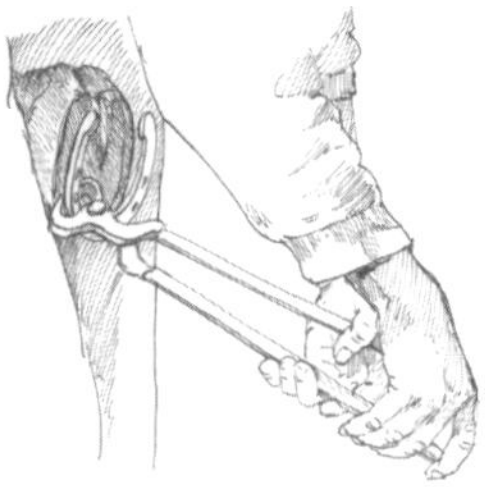

Step 2

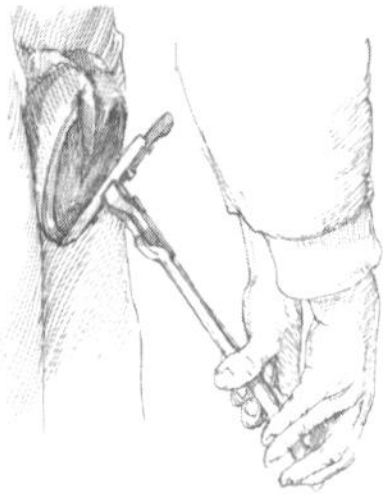

Step 3

Step 1. *Using a crease nail puller, pull a nail out to help loosen the shoe.*
Step 2. *Work down each branch of the shoe with alternate pulls, taking out each nail as you come to it.*
Step 3. *Pull the shoe.*

Close Nailed or Quicked

Given the large number of nails a farrier drives each year and the very narrow margin for error, it is inevitable that occasionally a shoeing nail may cause soreness. This typically shows up as marked lameness and a warm spot on the hoof within three days of the horse being shod. It is much more likely to occur when the feet are too short (from lost shoes, for example) and/or when the environment is wet. Call the farrier immediately. He'll remove the offending nail and may also need to remove the shoe to treat an abscess. You should also immediately check with your vet to be sure your horse is protected from tetanus.

Popped Clinches

If the clinches — the folded-over shank of the horseshoe nails where they exit the walls — have risen and stick up from the hoof wall, then the shoe is loose. Call your farrier.

Proper Care, With or Without Shoes

The first anti-horseshoeing movement arose in the late 1800s. A number of writers on horse care — such as Charles Page, John Wood, A. T. Fisher, and Jacob Ludlow — began blaming shoes for a wide variety of maladies. However, it was eventually realized that the root of most of these problems was not the shoes but poor stable conditions. Wood explains: "Whereas the hoof was intended by Nature to be nearly as hard as iron, man, in his attempts to improve upon Nature, does all in his power to soften it. . . . I therefore had the litter [bedding] removed by day [to completely air dry the stall floor every day] and . . . the horse's feet became tough . . . as oak." Wood and other horsemen then had no problems using unshod horses, even on paved city streets.

Common Hoof Wall Problems

Hoof wall problems are usually clearly visible, but because they come on slowly, they are often overlooked. Regular visits from a hoof care professional can help draw attention to these problems.

Cracks in the Hoof Wall

Horizontal cracks that run parallel with the coronet are due to abscesses that broke open at the coronet and drained. They usually need no attention and will grow down and out with the hoof wall. As the hoof wall typically grows about ¼ inch a month, you can easily estimate how long ago the abscess erupted by the distance the crack is from the coronet.

Sand cracks are numerous fine vertical cracks around the hoof wall that pass through only the outer surface of the hoof wall. These cracks and the weathering of the hoof wall make the hoof appear dried out and lacking in luster. Sand cracks (and dull, dry hooves) are due to frequent or extreme changes in moisture — much like the checking or weathering you see in exposed wood. The most effective remedy for sand cracks is maintaining a dry environment. A varnish-type hoof sealant can also be helpful. Moisturizing hoof dressings destroy the natural moisture gradient in the hoof wall and should be avoided.

Toe cracks are full-thickness vertical cracks due to overly long toes, breakover points that are too far forward, and/or damage to the coronary band above the crack that resulted in a weak area of wall being produced. A shorter toe and faster breakover will often eliminate the problem. However, if coronary band damage has occurred (it can typically be felt as an indentation just above the top of the hoof wall), cracks will be a chronic problem even with proper care. Find a good farrier and have your horse shod on a regular schedule.

Quarter cracks are full-thickness vertical cracks at the sides of the hoof that start at the coronet and come down. Quarter cracks may bleed. They are caused by overstressing of the hoof wall, often in conjunction with imbalanced or weak hooves. Balancing the hoof and shoeing with an eggbar and/or heartbar shoe can help stabilize the hoof and allow it to grow out solid again. Because quarter cracks are common on racehorses, you may be able to find a farrier who specializes in quarter crack repair at a nearby track.

Dull Walls

Dull and dry looking hoof walls may be due to a lack of essential fatty acids, in which case feeding flaxseed meal should help. Dull walls may also be due to arena footing modifiers such as salt; in this case, a varnish-type hoof coating may help. However, dull walls are most frequently due to exposure to moisture, urine, and manure — and it is the horse owner's responsibility to prevent this from happening.

Flares

Flares are those places where the hoof wall curves instead of being straight vertically. Flares occur when the wall is loaded with more weight than it can bear (or from a direction that it can't bear) without distorting. If the hoof is weak, flares will occur on both sides of the hoof equally. If there is a flare on just one side, then the hoof is being unevenly loaded; it is either out of balance or some gait abnormality is the cause. For example, flares to the insides of both front feet despite even wear on the shoes may be due to sore hips. Bring flares to the attention of your hoof care professional.

Hairy Hooves

When any part of the hoof wall breaks down into what looks like little bundles of hairs, it indicates that the feet have been exposed to an excessively alkaline environment. Most commonly this is the result of standing in urine or urine-soaked footing. The ammonia in urine is alkaline and dissolves the intertubular horn that holds the hairlike hoof tubules together. Find and eliminate areas where horses urinate and stand.

Run-Under Heels

With this condition, heels contact the ground too far forward, providing inadequate support for the foot. One cause of run-under heels is letting too much time elapse between shoeings. While there is no consistent cure, shoes can be set back to provide the proper, normal platform for the horse; cutting the heels down will move their point of support rearward; and wedge pads or wedge shoes can be used to reestablish the proper hoof angle.

Shelly Walls

Walls that come apart in layers or have cracks in the ground surface parallel with the white line are due to exposure to alkali. Shelly walls will progress to hairy hooves if not corrected. To prevent this, find and eliminate areas where horses urinate and stand.

Styrofoam Feet

Hooves that have become Styrofoam-like, airy, and weak are typically seen on show horses, which are are bathed (not just rinsed off) frequently. Soap is a milder alkali than urine, but frequent exposure to it, immediately followed by rapid drying (for example, in stalls bedded with wood chips), causes the hooves to lose much of their strength. A biotin and/or vitamin A deficiency might also be involved. To prevent or reverse this, avoid unnecessary bathing — just rinse off when possible — and be on the lookout for signs of a vitamin A or biotin deficiency (see the chart on page 6).

Wall–Sole Separation

Hooves that separate between the wall and sole, especially if it involves the entire hoof, have been exposed to moisture for prolonged periods. Horses who experience this problem typically spend many hours standing in a pond or stream. The cure is shoeing — to give the wall more strength — and fencing off the horse's access to such wet areas.

White Line Disease

More properly called *onychomycosis,* white line disease (WLD) does not affect the white line but rather the inner third (the white, unpigmented part) of the hoof wall. Hooves affected by WLD appear white, crumbly, and cheesy and often sound hollow when you tap on the hoof wall. The germs that cause WLD are everywhere, so it is not exposure to germs that causes it but, rather, a weakness of the feet that allows the germs to take hold. Treatment can be difficult and time consuming; it involves cutting away all the affected areas, frequent treatment with Merthiolate, keeping the horse in a very clean and dry environment, and nutrition that is low in carbohydrates and high in vitamin A. Consult with your hoof care professional if you suspect that your horse suffers from white line disease.

Sole and Frog Conditions

Sole and frog conditions may come on quickly, but they are often covered up with dirt. Be on the lookout for these conditions whenever you pick out a horse's hooves.

Abscesses

Abscesses are infections that are sealed off and produce pus, and therefore extreme pain. Abscesses may be due to puncture wounds, close shoeing nails, gravel embedded in the hoof, or even just moist footing that allows bacteria to gain access to sensitive tissues through the white line. Abscesses rarely occur when hooves are kept dry. In a typical case, the horse will go as quickly as overnight from being perfectly sound to being unwilling to bear any weight on the affected hoof. In this case, call your farrier or veterinarian immediately.

Your farrier or veterinarian should look for an entrance track and carefully open up the abscess to drain. Once the abscess is opened, soaking the hoof in a warm Epsom salt (magnesium sulfate) solution for 20 minutes at a time once or twice a day will help draw out the infection and promote faster healing. In order to draw out moisture, rather than add it, the Epsom salt solution must contain more Epsom salt than will dissolve in the water — at least 2 cups of Epsom salt per gallon of water. A few drops of betadine may also be added to the soaking solution. After all the pus has drained and the horse is sound, keep the foot absolutely dry for another three days to prevent reinfection.

Bruises

Horse with feet that are too short or soles that are too soft or thin often incur bruises on rocky ground. Bruises show up as red spots on the sole. However, they are not visible until at least a month after they occur, at which time they are no longer a problem. Immediate first aid for a bruised sole is to keep the horse off rocky ground and to tape cotton soaked in DMSO to the sole.

For prevention and long-term relief, shoes will help. Pads or boots may provide immediate temporary relief, but they trap moisture next to the foot and so do not cure the problem. Keep the feet dry. Painting the soles with turpentine or venice turpentine will help toughen and strengthen the soles.

Chalky Soles

Chalky, crumbling soles may be a symptom of a fungal infection, possibly caused by the horse standing in manure (which is not uncommon, even in the cleanest of barns). Prevent standing in bathroom areas if possible. Painting the soles with turpentine three times a week or more helps.

Flat Feet

Thoroughbreds and draft horses tend to be more susceptible to this condition. Damp footing will exacerbate the problem. Shoeing to give the hooves extra support and making sure the footing is kept clean and dry will usually correct the problem. If the soles are thin and tender, painting them daily with turpentine or venice turpentine is generally preferable to using pads, as pads trap moisture next to the hoof.

Stinky Feet

Hooves will naturally have some odor. However, if they are unusually smelly, treat them in the same manner as you would chalky soles (see page 27).

Thrush

Thrush is a smelly and greasy black discharge from the frog. It is generally thought to be caused by a filthy environment, but that is not the case. Some horses will not develop thrush when in constantly filthy footing, while other horses will get it even in a clean environment. Poor circulation is the most important cause of thrush. Horses who are lame in one leg will typically develop thrush in that leg because it gets less circulation.

Thrush in the collateral sulci can be cleaned with hydrogen peroxide and either left open to the air or treated with any of the commercial remedies. For thrush deep in the cleft of the frog, I prefer to first flush it out with hydrogen peroxide and cotton swabs, then pack the opening with zinc oxide ointment on a small piece of cotton ball. This should be changed every second day until the frog has grown out solid and healthy. Supplemental vitamin A may speed recovery and help prevent relapses.

Quick Tip

After you've handled a hoof infected with thrush, wash your hands with lemon juice. It will remove most of the smell.

Internal Hoof Diseases

With the exceptions of club foot and founder, internal hoof diseases cannot be seen directly but are found by observing signs of lameness, and by diagnosis by your vet.

Club Foot

Club foot is characterized by a hoof that has a toe angle of greater than 60 degrees and also grows more heel than toe when trimmed to less than 60 degrees. The hoof has a boxy look, with thin, straight walls at the quarters, a short frog, and most of the ground surface of the hoof in front of the center of rotation.

Club foot is not well understood and is rarely cured. However, centering the platform the horse stands on around the center of rotation (usually by using an eggbar shoe set well back from the toe) will often allow you to trim the hoof to 60 degrees or less and maintain that same angle until the next shoeing, while keeping the horse more comfortable.

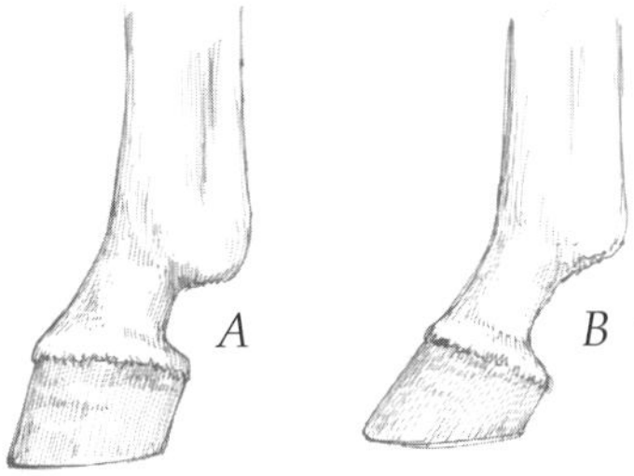

Club foot (A) compared with normal foot (B).

Laminitis

Laminitis is a disease that causes the weakening of the laminae (the attachment of the coffin bone to the hoof wall that supports the horse). Suspect laminitis if your horse walks as if on eggs, and especially if he appears uncomfortable turning sharply both to the right and to the left. Laminitis is consistently caused when a horse ingests an excess of carbohydrates, though there are many other causes that are not fully understood. Recent research indicates that fructans, produced by the action of sunlight on grass, may be the most likely carbohydrate to cause laminitis, so horses at risk of laminitis (those overweight even when on reduced rations) should be on pasture only at night, if at all, especially during the spring and fall when grass is lush and growing rapidly. If you have a horse at risk, discuss with your vet other possible preventive measures, such as muzzling or supplementing with 3 to 9 grams of magnesium per day.

Call your vet immediately if you see signs of laminitis or if your horse has broken into the feed bin and eaten too many carbohydrates. Because the laminae are weakened by laminitis, you must reduce stress on the laminae as much as possible in order to prevent founder. Exercise should be restricted, especially if pain medication is given. Gentle, even support for the whole bottom of the hoof (taping on styrofoam or standing on loose sand) will greatly reduce the stress on the laminae.

Horses that have laminitis due to endocrine problems, such as hypothyroidism or Cushing's syndrome, must be treated by the veterinarian, and they can be very difficult to keep healthy. Rather than having one episode of laminitis and resulting founder to recover from, they will instead have frequent, sometimes continual episodes of laminitis unless the endocrine problems can be managed with medications.

Founder

Founder is the typical result of laminitis. Founder results when the coffin bone rotates in relation to the hoof wall, tips down at the front, and/or sinks. Chronic founder results in distorted hooves — typically with high heels, a dished toe, and "founder rings" (hoof rings that are not parallel with the coronet but are closer to the coronet at the toe). Founder is best treated mechanically with therapeutic shoeing and trimming by your hoof care professional.

Foundered feet are much more susceptible to abscesses and infections. In these cases, sugardine (a thick paste of sugar and betadine), held against the hoof with bandages, is effective in cleaning up the infections.

Normal foot

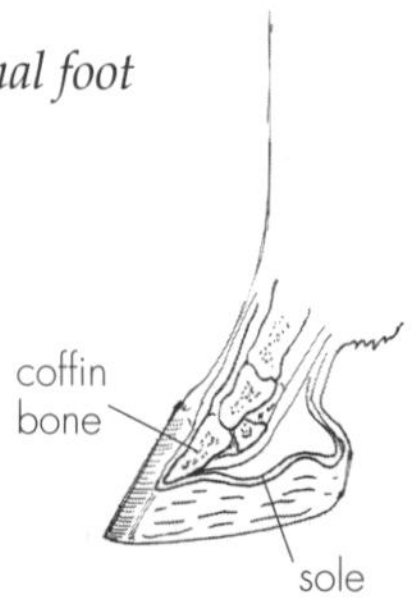

Foundered foot

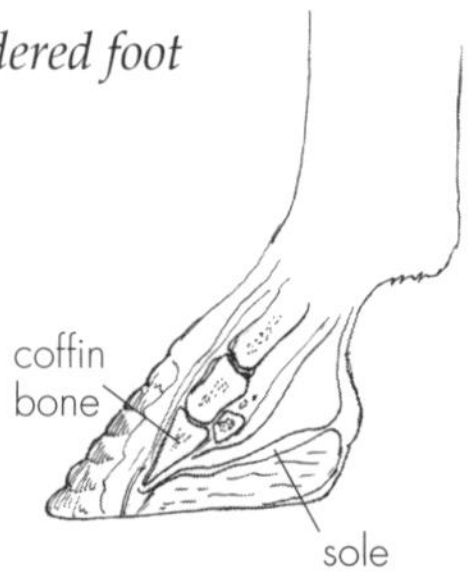

Because laminitis and founder are not yet fully understood, you are likely to hear completely opposing views on how to treat them. Some will recommend making the horse comfortable with bute, while others will say giving painkillers to a foundered horse is like giving painkillers to a football player with a broken leg — it makes him more comfortable, but it is going to cause him to do more damage to himself. Some will say to trim the heels low, and others say to shoe with wedge pads to raise the heels.

The most successful regimen I have seen includes restricting exercise; keeping the horse on soft, dry footing (clean, dry, loose sand or clean, deep wood shavings); frequent trimming toward more natural hoof/bone alignment (trimming the heels low and trimming the front of the toe back); and keeping the horse off all pain medication after the first 48 hours (as further overstress and damage may occur when the horse is not aware of the pain). Additional treatments I've found useful in some cases are resections, grooving the toe just under the coronet, and heartbar shoes. Each case is different and must be frequently monitored and adjusted by your hoof care professional. Until research can prove which method is most successful, find the best hoof care professional you can and let him do what he thinks is best.

Navicular Disease

Navicular disease is pain in the navicular region of the foot. Suspect it if your horse is short-strided and lands toe-first with both fore feet. Your vet can determine whether the cause is navicular disease.

Navicular disease may be due to tendinitis, bursitis, or arthritis. Shoeing can help by reducing stress to that area. Stress to the navicular area while standing or landing can be reduced by using a shoe that extends farther back (such as an eggbar shoe) and/or by raising the heel to increase the hoof angle (especially if the hoof itself is at an angle that is lower than normal). Stress to the navicular area while in motion can be reduced by decreasing the length of toe and/or by speeding up the breakover (with, for example, a rolled-toe shoe or a set-back shoe). Frequent mild exercise is helpful. Long periods kept in a stall alternated with hard work is very detrimental.

It is important to have the shoes reset on a regular schedule — the more often, the better — because that keeps the length of toe in check and reduces stress on the navicular area.

Working with Hoof Care Professionals, Vets, and Trainers

Everyone you ask for advice about horses has a different opinion. You can't take everyone's advice — it will just run you around in circles. Instead, find one expert in each area of horse care and stick with his or her advice.

Hoof care is not only a science, but also an art. There is no prescription or description detailed enough that will allow an inexperienced or untalented person to do a quality job. On the other hand, giving detailed instructions to an experienced and talented hoof care professional is simply a waste of his and your time. If you feel you have to give instructions, then you need to find a better hoof care professional.

It is wonderful for the horse and everyone concerned if the vet and hoof care professional can work in harmony. However, that only happens when each shows respect for the other's expertise. Any qualified and experienced hoof care professional should be more of an expert in shoeing and trimming than your vet. Follow your vet's advice on medicine and surgery; follow your hoof care professional's advice on trimming and shoeing. If the two professionals can work together smoothly, so much the better — but don't expect it. The only way they can possibly work together is if they communicate directly. If you relay veterinary instructions to your hoof care professional, you may not relay them completely or accurately. Even worse, this indirect method prevents your hoof care professional from making suggestions, asking questions, getting clarifications, and giving feedback to your vet. The Guild of Professional Farriers has a code of ethics for dealing with veterinarians that requires its members to communicate directly with the veterinarian on shared cases.

It is also very beneficial if your hoof care professional and trainer can work together. However, problems develop when one or another oversteps their area of expertise. You'll find your horse, and relationships, will benefit if you do not allow your trainer or vet to direct or prescribe shoeing and you do not allow your hoof care professional to prescribe training methods, surgery, or medications. Each person has their area of expertise — see that they don't step on each other's toes. If one of them says, "Tell your farrier/trainer/vet to do this," a good response is, "I hired him for his expertise, so I wouldn't tell him how to do his job any more than I would tell you how to do yours."